Dash Diet Cookbook 2021

A Complete Cooking Plan Full of Simple and
Tasty Recipes

Natalie Puckett

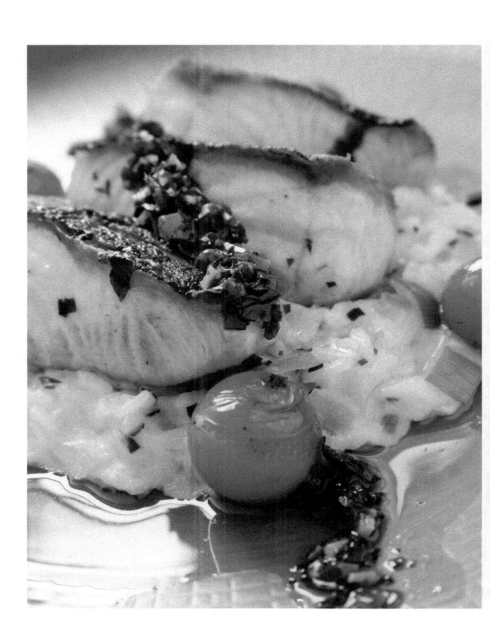

Table of Contents

Seafood-Stuffed Salmon Fillets

All out Time

Prep: 25 min. Heat: 20 min.

Makes

12 servings

Nutritional Facts: 1 stuffed filet: 454 calories, 27g fat (6g immersed fat), 123mg cholesterol, 537mg sodium, 9g starch (0 sugars, 0 filaments), and 41g protein.

Ingredients

1-1/2 cups cooked long-grain rice

1 bundle (8 ounces) impersonation crabmeat

2 tablespoons cream cheddar, relaxed

2 tablespoons margarine, dissolved

2 garlic cloves, minced

1/2 teaspoon each dried basil, marjoram, oregano, thyme, and rosemary, squashed

1/2 teaspoon celery seed, squashed

12 salmon filets (8 ounces each and 1-1/2 inches thick)

3 tablespoons olive oil

2 teaspoons dill weed

1-1/2 teaspoons salt

Direction

1.   Preheat stove to 400°. In an enormous bowl, join rice, crab, cream cheddar, spread, garlic, basil, marjoram, oregano, thyme, rosemary and celery seed.

2.   Cut a pocket on a level plane in each filet to inside 1/2 in. of the inverse side. Load up with stuffing blend; secure with toothpicks. Spot salmon on 2 lubed 15x10x1-in. heating skillet. Brush with oil; sprinkle with dill and salt.

3.   Bake 18-22 minutes or until fish just starts to chip effectively with a fork. Dispose of toothpicks before serving.

Classic Crab Boil

All out Time

Prep: 10 min. Cook: 30 min.

Makes

2 servings

Nutritional Facts: 1 crab: 245 calories, 3g fat (0 immersed fats), 169mg cholesterol, 956mg sodium, 2g starch (0 sugars, 0 fiber), 50g protein.

Ingredients

2 tablespoons mustard seed

2 tablespoons celery seed

1 tablespoon dill seed

1 tablespoon coriander seeds

1 tablespoon entire allspice

1/2 teaspoon entire cloves

4 cove leaves

Cheesecloth

8 quarts water

/4 cup salt

/4 cup lemon juice

teaspoon cayenne pepper

 entire live Dungeness crab (2 pounds each)

Melted margarine and lemon wedges

Directions

.   Place the initial seven fixings on a twofold thickness of
cheesecloth. Assemble corners of fabric to encase seasonings; tie
safely with string.

.   In an enormous stockpot, bring water, salt, lemon juice,
cayenne and flavor sack to a bubble. Utilizing tongs add crab to
stockpot; come back to a bubble. Decrease heat; stew, secured,
until shells turn splendid red, around 15 minutes.

.   Using tongs, expel crab from the pot. Dash under virus
water or dive into ice water. Present with dissolved margarine
and lemon wedges.

Foil-Packet Shrimp and Sausage Jambalaya

All out Time

Prep: 20 min. Heat: 20 min.

Makes

6 servings

1 parcel: 287 calories, 12g fat (4g immersed fat), 143mg cholesterol, 1068mg sodium, 23g starch (3g sugars, 2g fiber) 23g protein.

Ingredients

12 ounces completely cooked andouille wiener joins, cut into 1/2-inch cuts

12 ounces uncooked shrimp (31-40 for every pound), stripped and deveined

1 medium green pepper, slashed

1 medium onion, slashed

2 celery ribs, slashed

3 garlic cloves, minced

2 teaspoons Creole flavoring

1 can (14-1/2 ounces) fire-simmered diced tomatoes, depleted

1 cup uncooked moment rice

1 can (8 ounces) tomato sauce

1/2 cup chicken juices

Directions

1. Preheat broiler to 425°. In an enormous bowl, join all fixings. Partition blend among 6 lubed 18x12-in. Bits of substantial foil. Crease foil around blend and pleat edges to seal, framing bundles; place on a heating sheet. Prepare until shrimp turn pink and rice is delicate, 20-25 minutes.

Lemony Scallops with Angel Hair Pasta

Complete Time

Prep/Total Time: 25 min.

Makes

4   servings

Nourishment Facts: 1-1/2 cups: 404 calories, 13g fat (2g soaked fat), 27mg cholesterol, 737mg sodium, 48g starch (4g sugars, 6g fiber), and 25g protein.

Ingredients

8 ounces uncooked multigrain holy messenger hair pasta

3 tablespoons olive oil, separated

1 pound ocean scallops, tapped dry

2 cups cut radishes (around 1 pack)

2 garlic cloves, cut

1/2 teaspoon squashed red pepper chips 6 green onions, daintily cut 1/2 teaspoon legitimate salt

1 tablespoon ground lemon get-up-and-go 1/4 cup lemon juice

Directions

1.   In a 6-qt. stockpot, cook pasta as per bundle bearings; channel and come back to the pot.

2.   Meanwhile, in a huge skillet, heat 2 tablespoons oil over medium-high warmth; singe scallops in clusters until misty and edges are brilliant darker, around 2 minutes for every side. Expel from skillet; keep warm.

3.   In a similar skillet, saute radishes, garlic and pepper chips in residual oil until radishes are delicate, 2-3 minutes. Mix in green onions and salt; cook 1 moment. Add to pasta; hurl to consolidate. Sprinkle with lemon pizzazz and juice. Top with scallops to serve.

Pan-Seared Salmon with Dill Sauce

Complete Time

Prep/Total Time: 25 min.

Makes

4 servings

Nourishment Facts: 1 salmon filet with 1/4 cup sauce: 366 calories, 25g fat (4g soaked fat), 92mg cholesterol, 349mg sodium, 4g starch (3g sugars, 0 fibers), 31g protein. Diabetic trades: 4 lean meat, 2-1/2 fat.

Ingredients:

1 tablespoon canola oil

4 salmon filets (6 ounces each)

1 teaspoon Italian flavoring

1/4 teaspoon salt

1/2 cup decreased fat plain yogurt

1/4 cup decreased fat mayonnaise

1/4 cup finely hacked cucumber

teaspoon cut crisp dill

Directions

.	In a huge skillet, heat oil over medium-high warmth. Sprinkle salmon with Italian flavoring and salt. A spot in skillet, kin side down. Lessen warmth to medium. Cook until fish just tarts to drop effectively with a fork, around 5 minutes on each ide.

2.	Meanwhile, in a little bowl, join yogurt, mayonnaise, cucumber, and dill. Present with salmon.

Chicken Bruschetta

SmartPoints value: Green plan - 1SP, Blue plan - 1SP, Purple plan - 1SP

Total Time: 20 min, Prep time: 10 min, Cooking time: 10 min, Serves: 4

Nutritional value: Calories - 187, Carbs – 4.4g, Fat - 7g, Protein – 27.3g

When the weather is heating up, I mostly crave for fresh and light meals other than rich and comforting.

My most recently found new love when it comes to dessert is this deliciously prepared Italian Chicken Bruschetta. It's just so simple, simply made with fresh tomatoes, basil, and garlic. I've tried it several times, and one sweet thing about it is the refreshing flavors. There is just something about the way the fresh and juicy tomato works together with the bright basil and bold garlic.

While preparing, I like to add some grilled chicken breast to it as a lean protein. If you've noticed, I do more of chicken breast, yes, because it is low in points, and it's a perfect way of adding protein to my meal without getting over budget with my points.

Ingredients

Chicken breast (skinless, boneless) - 1 lb

Large Roma tomatoes (finely diced) - 2 pieces

Basil (finely chopped, fresh) - 1/4 cup

Garlic (minced) - 2 cloves

Olive oil (1 tbsp plus 1 tsp)

Balsamic Vinegar (1/2 tsp)

Parsley (dried) - 1 tsp

Oregano (dried) - 1 tsp

Pepper and Salt to taste

Instructions

1.	After cutting the chicken breasts into four equal-sized fillets, season each of the side of the chicken with the parsley, oregano and salt and pepper.

2.	Over medium-high heat, heat one teaspoon of olive oil in a medium-sized, nonstick skillet. For 4-5 minutes, cook as you turn each side until the chicken is entirely cooked and browned.

3.	Remove from heat and cover with a lid to allow it to sit for about 5 minutes.

4.	Make bruschetta by mixing tomatoes, olive oil, garlic, basil, balsamic vinegar, and pepper and salt in a bowl.

5.	Put the chicken breast on a plate and top each of them with about ¼ cup of the bruschetta. Then drizzle on some extra balsamic if you so desire.

6.   You can also make a sandwich with fresh Italian bread and little creamy goat cheese. The flavor is so bold and mouthwatering.

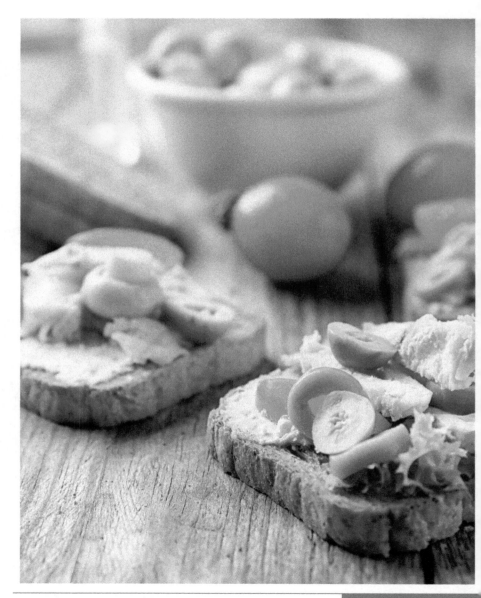

Lemon Chicken with Broccoli

SmartPoints value: Green plan - 3SP, Blue plan - 1SP, Purple plan - 1SP

Total Time: 30 min, Prep time: 15 min, Cooking time: 15 min, Serves: 4

Nutritional value:

Calories - 176.6, Carbs - 8.4g, Fat - 2.0g, Protein - 32.3g

The whole family will love this fantastic weeknight dinner, and it's ready in just 30 minutes. To ensure that the chicken cooks quickly and evenly, you should slice it thinly. Cover the pan when cooking the broccoli to help build up steam, bathing the florets with heat. It will allow tops that aren't in contact with the hot pan to cook properly. You will need one small to medium head of broccoli to get enough florets and one lemon to yield enough zest and juice for this entrée.

Ingredients

All-purpose flour - 2 Tbsp

Black pepper - ¼ tsp (freshly ground)

Fat-free, reduced-sodium chicken broth - 1½ cup(s) (divided)

Fresh lemon juice - 1 Tbsp

Fresh parsley - 2 Tbsp (chopped)

Lemon zest - 2 tsp, or more to taste*

Minced Garlic - 2 tsp

Olive oil - 2 tsp

Table salt - ½ tsp (divided)

Uncooked chicken breast(s) -12 oz, thinly sliced (boneless, skinless)

Uncooked broccoli - 2½ cup(s), small florets

Instructions

1.   On a clean plate, mix 1 1/2 Tbsp of flour, 1/4 tsp of salt, and pepper, then add chicken and turn to coat.

2.   Put a large nonstick skillet over medium-high heat and pour the oil in for heating.

3.   Add the chicken and cook, turning as needed, until it is lightly browned and cooked through, about 5 minutes; remove to a plate.

4.   Put one cup of broth and Garlic in the same skillet, then boil over high heat, scraping up browned bits from the bottom of the pan with a wooden spoon.

5.   Add the broccoli, then cover and cook for 1 minute.

6.   Stir the remaining 1/2 cup broth, 1/2 Tbsp flour, and 1/4 tsp salt together in a small cup, then add to the skillet and bring its content to a simmer over low heat.

7.   Cover the skillet and cook until the broccoli is crisp-tender and the sauce thickens slightly.

8.   Stir in the chicken and lemon zest, then heat through.

9.   Remove the skillet from heat, and stir in the parsley and lemon juice, then toss to coat.

Chicken and Fennel in Rosemary-wine Broth

SmartPoints value: Green plan - 4SP, Blue plan - 2SP, Purple plan - 2SP

Total Time: 40 min, Prep time: 18 min, Cooking time: 22 min. Serves: 4

Nutritional value: Calories - 121.5, Carbs - 10.5g, Fat - 6.3g, Protein - 26.0g

If you are looking for a dish that will tickle your belly on a chilly night, this rustic Italian entrée is perfect, and since you will cook it in one skillet, that **Makes** it easy to fix in your vegetable. You should first sear the chicken to produce an excellent brown exterior. You can then sauté the fennel and onion in the flavorful drippings left in the skillet. They will mix and become sweetened as they cook.

Return the chicken and any accumulated juices to the skillet to finish cooking.

Ingredients

All-purpose flour - 5 tsp (divided)

Black pepper - ⅛ tsp, or to taste (freshly ground)

Canned chicken broth - 14½ oz

Minced Garlic - 2 tsp

Olive oil - 1 Tbsp, extra-virgin (divided)

Red/white wine - 1/4 cup

Rosemary - 1¼ tsp, fresh (chopped)

Table salt - ½ tsp, or to taste

Uncooked chicken breast(s) - 1 pound(s), cut into bite-size chunks (boneless, skinless)

Uncooked fennel bulb(s) - 1 pound(s)

Uncooked red onion(s) - 1 small (chopped)

Instructions

1.   Trim the stalk from fennel to quarter bulb(s) lengthwise and then slice in a cross-like manner into small pieces. Reserve the fronds for garnish (about 3 cups fennel will be available).

2.   Put the chicken on a plate and sprinkle it with rosemary, then sprinkle it with 4 tsp flour and toss to coat.

3.   Add 1 tsp of oil to a large nonstick skillet and heat over medium-high heat.

4.   Add the chicken and cook, occasionally turning with tongs, until it is lightly brown.

5.   Transfer the chicken to a clean plate (cooking is partial at this point).

6.   Heat the remaining 2 tsp oil in the same skillet over medium-high heat and add fennel and onion; sauté until it

becomes lightly brown and almost tender.

7.   Add wine and Garlic, then reduce the heat to low and simmer, stirring the bottom of the pan to scrape up browned bits, until most of the wine has evaporated.

8.   Stir the broth together with the remaining 1 tsp flour in a small bowl and then stir into skillet.

9.   Add salt and pepper, then increase the heat to high and bring it to a boil. Reduce the heat to medium-low and simmer for another 1 minute.

10.   Add the chicken and cook, often tossing until the chicken cooks through. Garnish with reserved chopped fennel fronds and serve.

You can serve it with crusty whole-grain bread, or over rice, to mop up all of the broth.

If you prefer not to use wine in this recipe, you can substitute with one tablespoon of red or white wine vinegar and three tablespoons of water.

Chicken Cordon Bleu

SmartPoints value: Green plan - 6SP, Blue plan - 4SP, Purple plan - 4SP

Total Time: 46 min, Prep time: 11 min, Cooking time: 35 min, Serves: 4

Nutritional value: Calories - 357.9, Carbs - 12.7g, Fat - 16.9g, Protein - 36.7g

Cordon bleu was a commonly served dish at dinner-parties in the sixties. Preparing it is simple: You sandwich a layer of ham and cheese between thin medallions of chicken or veal, then you sauté it.

Here, I have created a light version of the recipe to use a single layer of chicken rolled around the filling to make an elegant presentation.

Prepare this dish the next time you have guests and add some greens to the plate: either roasted broccolini, asparagus, or haricot vert (thin French green beans) will do just fine.

Ingredients

All-purpose flour - 4 Tbsp

Black pepper - ⅛ tsp (or to taste), freshly ground

Cornflake crumbs - ½ cup(s)

Lean ham (cooked) - 4 slice(s), (about 2 oz. total)

Egg(s) - 1 large, lightly beaten

Ground nutmeg - ⅛ tsp

Parmesan cheese - 2 Tbsp, freshly grated

Reduced-sodium chicken broth - ½ cup(s)

Swiss cheese - 2 oz (4 thin slices), low-fat

Table salt - ½ tsp

Table wine - 1 Tbsp, Madeira

Uncooked chicken breast(s) -1 pound(s), (4 breasts, 1/4 pound each), pounded to ¼-inch thickness (boneless, skinless)

2% reduced-fat milk - ½ cup(s)

Instructions

1.   Spray a baking sheet with nonstick spray while you preheat the oven to 400°F.

2.   Place one half of a chicken breast on a work surface and top it with one slice of the ham, then one slice of the Swiss cheese.

3.   Roll it up in a jelly-roll style, and secure with a toothpick. Repeat the process with the remaining chicken, ham, and cheese.

4.   Make a mixture of two tablespoons of flour, one-quarter teaspoon of salt, and ground pepper on a sheet of wax paper.

5.   Place the egg and the cornflake crumbs in separate shallow bowls.

5.   Taking it one at a time, coat the chicken rolls lightly, first with the flour mixture, and then dip it into the egg for a single layer coat.

7.   Coat the rolls with the cornflake crumbs, and place them on the baking sheet (discard any leftover flour mixture, egg, and cornflake bits).

8.   Spray the chicken rolls lightly with nonstick spray. Bake until the temperature of the rolls reaches 160°F, 30–35 minutes.

9.   To prepare the sauce, mix the milk, the broth, the Madeira, nutmeg, the remaining two tablespoons of flour, the remaining 1/4 teaspoon of salt, and another grinding of the pepper in a medium-sized saucepan.

10.   Whisk until it is smooth and cook over medium heat, continually whisking until it becomes thick in about 6 minutes.

11.   Remove the sauce from the heat and stir in the Parmesan cheese, then cover to keep it warm.

12.   When the chicken rolls are ready, drizzle them with the sauce and serve them immediately.

Peanut Butter Sandwich Snacks

SmartPoints value: Green plan - 3SP, Blue plan - 3SP, Purple plan - 3SP
Total Time: 5 min, Prep time: 5 min, Serves: 1
Nutritional value: Calories - 327, Carbs - 30g, Fat - 17.9g, Protein - 15.0g

Ingredients

Peanut butter (powdered) - 1 Tbsp

Water - 2¼ tsp

Crispbread, Whole Grain (34 degrees) - 6 crackers, or similar product

Chocolate syrup - 1½ tsp

Sprinkles - ¼ tsp, nonpareil

Instructions

1.   Mix the powdered peanut butter and water in a clean small bowl and stir until it becomes smooth.

2.   Spread the peanut butter evenly over three crackers and top it with the remaining three crackers biscuit or bread.

3.   Take half a teaspoon of chocolate syrup and spread it over half the top of each cracker sandwich — top chocolate syrup with sprinkles.

Peanut Butter Apple Slices

SmartPoints value: Green plan - 4SP, Blue plan - 4SP, Purple plan - 4SP

Total time: 10 min, Prep time: 10 min, Serves: 4

Nutritional value: Calories - 218, Carbs – 31.3g, Fat – 8.1g, Protein – 11.6g

Having a healthy snack ready in about 10 minutes is a thing of joy for me. Peanut butter apple slices are just what fits into the picture of a healthy quick, nutritious snack. This apple slice is a simple and easy meal rich in protein and fiber. It is topped with peanut butter and decorated with chocolate chips and slivered almonds.

Ingredients

Large apples - 2 pieces

Powdered peanut butter (reconstituted) - 1/2 cup

Semi-sweet chocolate chips - 2 tbsp

Slivered almonds - 2 tbsp

Pecans (chopped) - 2 tbsp

Instructions

1.   Remove the core of the apple using a small paring knife or an apple corer

2. Slice the apples into thick rings.

3. Add the peanut butter on the apple slices.

4. Use chips and nuts for top-up

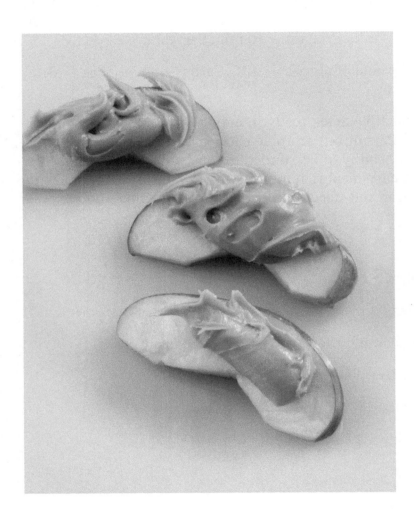

Baked Plantains

SmartPoints value: Green plan - 5SP, Blue plan - 5SP, Purple plan   -   5SP
Total time: 40 min, Prep time: 5 min, Cooking time: 35min, Serves: 2
Nutritional value: Calories - 184, Carbs - 47g, Fat – 0.5g, Protein -   2g

Baked plantain is just as healthy as it is tasty. The plantain is full of good for your **Ingredients**.

Ingredients

Very overripe plantains (2 medium-sized)

Misting spray (Olive oil)

Salt to taste

Instructions

1.   On a preheated oven of 350 degrees, line a baking sheet with a silicone mat or parchment paper and spray with olive oil or non-fat cooking spray.

2.   Thinly slice plantains and place them on the baking sheet evenly, then lightly mist with olive oil or the non-fat cooking spray and sprinkle with a bit of salt.

3.   For about 30-35 minutes, cook in the oven flipping once about halfway through until they become golden and mostly crisp.

Baked plantains are easy to prepare and very firm. They taste sweeter when overly ripe, and firmer when they are not as ripe. Feel free to choose your style of plantain.

Strawberries & Cream Chocolate Cookie Sandwich

SmartPoints value: Green plan - 3SP, Blue plan - 3SP, Purple plan - 3SP

Total time: 5 min, Prep time: 5 min, Serves: 1

Nutritional value: Calories - 280, Carbs - 37g, Fat - 12g, Protein - 5g

Ingredients

Topping (lite whipped) - 2 Tbsp Strawberries (hulled, sliced) - 1 medium

Graham cracker(s) (chocolate variety) - 2 square(s)

Instructions

.   Scoop whipped topping onto one square-shaped graham cracker.

2.   Top it with sliced strawberries and place another cracker on top of that.

Mini chocolate chip cookies

SmartPoints value: Green plan - 1SP, Blue plan - 1SP, Purple plan - 1SP

Total time: 26 min, Prep time: 10 min, Cooking time: 6 min, Serves: 48

Nutritional value: Calories - 113.7, Carbs - 16.4g, Fat - 5.9g, Protein - 0.6g

Ingredients

Butter (salted, softened) - 2 Tbsp

Canola oil - 2 tsp

Brown sugar (packed, dark-variety) - ½ cup(s)

Vanilla extract - 1 tsp

Table salt - ⅛ tsp

Egg white(s) - 1 large

All-purpose flour - ¾ cup(s)

Baking soda - ¼ tsp

Chocolate chips (semi-sweet) - 3 oz, about 1/2 cup

Instructions

1.   Prepare the oven by preheating it to 375°F.

2.   Mix the butter, oil, and sugar in a medium bowl.

3.   Add vanilla and egg white, then mix thoroughly to combine. Toss in some salt to taste.

4.   Mix the flour and baking soda in a small bowl and stir them into the batter.

5.   Add the chocolate chips to the batter and stir to distribute evenly throughout.

6.   Put forty-eight half-teaspoons of dough onto two large nonstick baking sheets. Leave small spaces between the cookies.

7.   Bake the cookies until they become golden around the edges; about 4 to 6 minutes.

8.   Cool the baked cookies on a wire rack.

Chocolate-Peppermint Thins

SmartPoints value: Green plan - 3SP, Blue plan - 3SP, Purple plan   -   3SP
Total Time: 1hr 16 min, Prep time: 15 min, Cooking time: 5 min, Serves: 16
Nutritional value: Calories - 175, Carbs – 21g, Fat – 5g, Protein – 7g
My homemade chocolate peppermint thin comes with a splash of peppermint extract, and divine copycat thin mint cookies to satisfy my cravings

Ingredients

Chocolate chunk (coarsely chopped) - 3½ oz

Chocolate wafer(s) (thin variety) - 16 item(s)

Candy cane (finely crushed) - 1 oz

Instructions

1.   Arrange a large baking sheet with parchment or paper wax and line cookies close together in a single layer.

2.   At 5 seconds interval, melt chocolate in a microwavable bowl and stir between each interval until all but one or two pieces melted, then remove from microwave and stir until fully dissolved.

3.   Put the melted chocolate in a plastic bag and cut off a corner; in a zig-zag pattern, pipe the chocolate over cookies and

sprinkle with the crushed candy cane, keep it refrigerated until its set for at least an hour or overnight. Serve as desired (1 cookie per serving)

Chocolate-Dipped Baby Bananas

SmartPoints value: Green plan - 3SP, Blue plan - 3SP, Purple plan - 3SP

Total time: 20 min, Prep time: 5 min, Cooking time: --, Serves: 12

Nutritional value: Calories - 210, Carbs – 31.2g, Fat – 1g, Protein – 5.4g

Chocolate-dipped baby bananas are just perfect for casual parties for both kids and adults. With the banana and chocolate combination, it's so irresistible. Alternatively, you can replace baby bananas with four regular bananas cut crosswise into thirds.

Ingredients

Baby-variety banana (peeled) - 12 small

Chocolate (semisweet, chopped) - 3 oz

Butter (unsalted) - ¾ tsp

Coconut (shredded, unsweetened) - 2 tbsp

Instructions

1.   Place large baking sheet with wax paper and insert wooden craft stick in one end of each banana.

2.   Mix butter and chocolate in a medium microwave bowl, then microwave on high heat for about 1minute.

3.   Taking one banana after another spoon the chocolate over the bananas cover, and sprinkle it with coconut while it is on a baking sheet. Keep it refrigerated until the chocolate sets in about 15 minutes.

4.   Serve as desired (1 banana per serving)

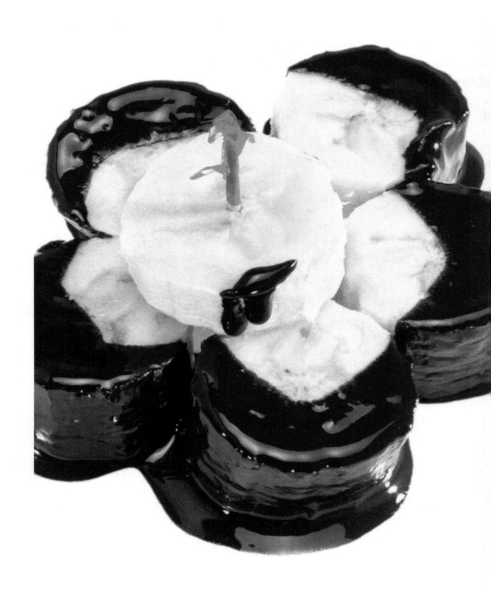

Mango Salsa

SmartPoints value: Green plan - 0SP, Blue plan - 0SP, Purple plan - 0SP
Total time: 15 min, Prep time: 15 min, Cooking time: 0 min, Serves: 4
Nutritional value: Calories – 71, Carbs – 17.7g, Fat – 0.5g, Protein – 1.3g

The mango salsa is a great snack full of fruits and veggies. Although salsa goes well with chips, it doesn't mean that you can use it for other things. However, it's an excellent topper for fish, chicken, and even salads.

Ingredients

Large mango (peeled and diced) - 1 item

Red onion (finely chopped) - 1/2

Red bell pepper (chopped) - 1 cup

Jalapeno pepper (seeded and chopped) - (1 small piece)

Garlic (minced) - 2 cloves

Lime juice - 1 cup

Pinch of salt (add to taste)

Instructions

1.   Put all the **Ingredients** in a bowl and season as desired with salt.

2.   This mouthwatering sweet and savory salsa awakens your taste buds with delicious flavors. It is fresh, light, and loaded with antioxidants that make it a great pair with tortilla chips.

Watermelon Aguas Frescas

SmartPoints value: 3SP
Total time: 5 min, Prep time: 5 min, Serves – 4
Nutritional value: Calories - 57, Carbs - 14g, Fat - 0g, Protein - 1g

Ingredients

Watermelon (seedless, ripe; make sure it's nice and sweet) - 4 cups cubed

Sugar (honey or agave nectar as an alternative) - 1 tbsp (or to taste)

Water - 3 cups

Lime juice (fresh) - 2-3 tsps.

Mint (fresh) for garnish, if you desire

Instructions

1.   Put the cubed watermelon in a blender and add 1-1/2 cups of the water, the lime juice, and the sugar. Blend everything at high speed until smooth.

2.   Sieve the liquid blend through a medium strainer into a large pitcher (or bowl).

3.   Pour in the remaining 1-1/2 cups of water and stir.

4.   Chill in a refrigerator for 1 hour or longer, depending on the temperature you like.

5. Drop a few cubes of ice in a glass and pour in the watermelon agua fresca.

6. Add a mint sprig to garnish if you desire.

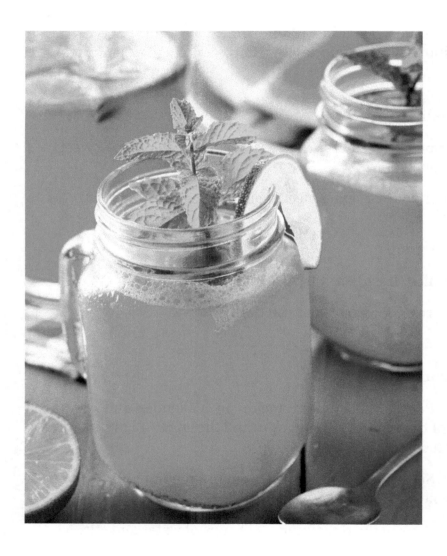

Chocolate Peanut Butter Banana Protein Shake

SmartPoints value: 6SP

Total time: 5 min, Prep time: 5 min, Serves: 1

Nutritional value: Calories - 299, Carbs - 29.6g, Fat - 6.1g, Protein - 36.2g

This drink provides a fast, healthy, and delicious way to begin your day, packed with protein to help keep you satisfied until lunchtime.

Ingredients

Cottage cheese (non-fat) - 1/2 cup

Peanut Butter Flour (PB2) - 2 tablespoons

Chocolate protein powder - 1 scoop

Banana (frozen) - 1/2 finger

A handful of ice cubes

Sweetener - to taste (You may not need this if your protein powder already has sweetener in it)

Instructions

1.   Mix all the **Ingredients** in a blender and process until you get a smooth mixture.

2.   You can add more ice cubes to give a thicker consistency to the protein shake.

3.   You can use less ice if you want your drink to be thinner. Add more water.

Skinny Pina Colada

SmartPoints - 7SP

Total time: 5 min, Prep time: 5 min, Serves: 1

Nutritional value: Calories - 183, Carbs - 11g, Fat - 0.5g, Protein - 9.5g

Ingredients

Vanilla protein powder with about 100 calories per 1-ounce serving (natural) - 3 tablespoons

Crushed pineapple packed in juice (canned, not drained) - 1/4 cup

White rum - 1 -1/2 ounces

Coconut extract - 1/8 teaspoon

Crushed ice, about eight ice cubes - 1 cup

Instructions

1.   Put all the **Ingredients** in a blender.

2.   Pour in half a cup of water, and blend at high speed until it is smooth.

Spindrift Grapefruit

SmartPoints value: 1SP

Serving size - 355ml

Nutritional value: Calories - 17, Carbs - 4g, Fat - 0g, Protein - 0g

Spindrift is America's first sparkling water fruit drink.

The several varieties of the drink are all created from sparkling water and real squeezed fruits.

Aside from the grapefruit variety, the other types you can enjoy with your meal include blackberry, cucumber, lemon, raspberry lime, orange mango, strawberry, half & half, and cranberry raspberry.

Ingredients

The **Ingredients** of Grapefruit drink include grapefruit juice, lemon juice, orange juice.

Popcorn

It's a tasty, rather low-calorie snack that can be ready to eat in under 10 minutes. It's perfect if you're craving something a little salty.

Nutritional Facts

servings per container	5
Prep Total	**10 min**
Serving Size	8
Amount per serving **Calories**	**0%**
	% Daily Value
Total Fat 3g	**20%**
Saturated Fat 4g	32%
Trans Fat 2g	2%
Cholesterol	**2%**
Sodium 110mg	**0.2%**
Total Carbohydrate 21g	**50%**
Dietary Fiber 9g	1%
Total Sugar 1g	1%
Protein 1g	
Vitamin C 7mcg	17%
Calcium 60mg	1%
Iron 7mg	10%
Potassium 23mg	21%

Ingredient & Process

Place 2 tablespoons of olive oil and ¼ Cup popcorn in a large saucepan.

Cover with a lid, and cook the popcorn over a medium flame, ensuring that you are shaking constantly. Just when you think that it's not working, keep on enduring for another minute or two, and the popping will begin.

When the popping stops, take off from the heat and place in a large bowl.

Add plenty of salt to taste, and if desired, dribble in ¼ Cup to ½ Cup of melted coconut oil. If you are craving sweet popcorn, add some maple syrup to the coconut oil, about ½ Cup, or to taste.

5 Minutes or Less Vegan Snacks

Here's a list of basically 'no-preparation required' vegan snack ideas that you can munch on anytime:

Nutritional Facts

servings per container	5
Prep Total	**10 min**
Serving Size	8
Amount per serving **Calories**	**0%**
	% Daily Value
Total Fat 20g	**190%**
Saturated Fat 2g	32%
Trans Fat 1g	2%
Cholesterol	**2%**
Sodium 70mg	**0.2%**
Total Carbohydrate 32g	**150%**
Dietary Fiber 8g	1%
Total Sugar 1g	1%
Protein 3g	
Vitamin C 7mcg	17%
Calcium 210mg	1%
Iron 4mg	10%
Potassium 25mg	20%

Ingredients and Process

Trail mix: nuts, dried fruit, and vegan chocolate pieces.

Fruit pieces with almond butter, peanut butter or vegan chocolate spread

Frozen vegan cake, muffin, brownie or slice that you made on the weekend

Vegetable sticks (carrots, celery, and cucumber etc.) with a Vegan Dip (homemade or store-bought) such as hummus or beetroot dip. (Careful of the store-bought **Ingredients** though).

Smoothie - throw into the blender anything you can find (within limits!) such as soy milk, coconut milk, rice milk, almond milk, soy yogurt, coconut milk yogurt, cinnamon, spices, sea salt, berries, bananas, cacao powder, vegan chocolate, agave nectar, maple syrup, chia seeds, flax seeds, nuts, raisins, sultanas... What you put into your smoothie is up to you, and you can throw it all together in less than 5 minutes!

Crackers with avocado, soy butter, and tomato slices, or hummus spread.

Packet chips (don't eat them too often). There are many vegan chip companies that make kale chips, corn chips, potato chips, and vegetable chips, so enjoy a small bowl now and again.

Fresh Fruit

The health benefits of eating fresh fruit daily should not be minimized. So, make sure that you enjoy some in-season fruit as one of your daily vegan snacks.

Nutritional Facts

servings per container	10
Prep Total	**10 min**
Serving Size	5/5
Amount per serving **Calories**	**1%**
	% Daily Value
Total Fat 24g	**2%**
Saturated Fat 8g	3%
Trans Fat 4g	2%
Cholesterol	**2%**
Sodium 10mg	**22%**
Total Carbohydrate 7g	**54%**
Dietary Fiber 4g	1%
Total Sugar 1g	1%
Protein 1g	24
Vitamin C 2mcg	17%
Calcium 270mg	15%
Iron 17mg	20%
Potassium 130mg	2%

Ingredients:

Chop your favorite fruit and make a fast and easy fruit salad, adding some squeezed orange juice to make a nice juicy dressing.
Serve with some soy or coconut milk yogurt or vegan ice-cream if desired, and top with some tasty walnuts or toasted slithered almonds to make it a sustaining snack.

Vegan Brownie

Nutritional Facts

servings per container	3
Prep Total	**10 min**
Serving Size	7
Amount per serving **Calories**	**20%**
	% Daily Value
Total Fat 3g	**22%**
Saturated Fat 22g	8%
Trans Fat 17g	21%
Cholesterol	**20%**
Sodium 120mg	**70%**
Total Carbohydrate 30g	**57%**
Dietary Fiber 4g	8%
Total Sugar 10g	8%
Protein 6g	
Vitamin C 1mcg	1%
Calcium 20mg	31%
Iron 2mg	12%
Potassium 140mg	92%

Ingredients:

1/2 cup non-dairy butter melted

5 tablespoons cocoa

1 cup granulated sugar

3 teaspoons Ener-G egg replacer

1/4 cup water

1 teaspoon vanilla

3/4 cup flour

1 teaspoon baking powder

1/2 teaspoon salt

1/2 cup walnuts (optional)

Instructions:

1. Heat oven to 350°. Prepare an 8" x 8" baking pan with butter or canola oil.

2. Combine butter, cocoa, and sugar in a large bowl.

3. Mix the egg replacer and water in a blender until frothy.

4. Add to the butter mixture with vanilla. Add the flour, baking powder, and salt, and mix thoroughly.

5. Add the walnuts if desired. Pour the batter into the pan, and spread evenly.

6. Bake for 40 to 45 minutes, or until a toothpick inserted comes out clean.

Barley, Grape Tomato and Arugula Sauté

SmartPoints value: Green plan - 3SP, Blue plan - 3SP, Purple plan - 1SPTotal time: 50 min, Prep time: 10 min, Cooking time: 40 min, Serves: 4
Nutritional value: Calories - 82.8, Carbs - 4.8g Fat - 7.2g, Protein - 1.2g
This grain and vegetable side dish is colourful and sweet with a peppery bite.
Toss in some yellow grape tomatoes to add even more colour.

Ingredients

Water - 1¼ cup(s)

Table salt - ¾ tsp, divided

Pearl barley (uncooked) - ½ cup(s)

Olive oil (extra-virgin) - 1½ tsp, divided

Tomatoes (grape) - 1½ cup(s), halved

Minced garlic - 1½ tsp

Black pepper (freshly ground) - ¼ tsp

Arugula (baby leaves) - 3 cup(s)

Lemon zest (finely grated) - ¼ tsp (or to taste)

Instructions

1.   Stir half tsp of salt into a small saucepan of water and bring it to a boil. Add barley to it and cover; reduce the heat to low and cook until the water is absorbed and the barley is tender but still has a nice bite to it; about 30-35 minutes. Remove the saucepan from the heat and set it aside.

2.   Apply heat to one teaspoon of oil in a medium nonstick skillet over medium-high heat. Add the tomatoes and garlic, then sauté it until the tomatoes start to soften and release their juices; about 1-2 minutes.

3.   Put in more barley, the remaining one-quarter teaspoon of salt and

pepper, and reduce the heat to medium and cook, stirring it until the tomatoes soften further and the grain absorbs tomato liquid; about 2-3 minutes.

4.   Stir in the arugula and toss it over medium heat until it wilts; about 30 seconds.

5.   Remove the dish from the heat and stir in the remaining half teaspoon of oil and lemon zest.

Note: You can reheat this recipe the next day, and it will still taste great. Alternatively, you can serve it as a cold salad. Allow it come to room temperature and then toss it, adding just a bit of red wine or balsamic vinegar.

Creamy Mushroom and Chicken Stew Crockpot

SmartPoints value: Green plan - 2SP, Blue plan - 2SP, Purple plan - 2SP
Total Time: 4hr 20min, Prep time: 10 min, Cooking time: 4hr 10mins,
Serves: 4
Nutritional value: Calories – 278, Carbs – 24.2g, Fat – 4.2g, Protein – 32g

The mushroom and chicken stew crockpot is a fantastic low-calorie dinner idea. It's a healthy and easy slow cooker recipe with   great   taste.

Ingredients

Chicken breast (skinless) - 1 lb

Baby portabella mushroom (sliced) - 8 oz

Onion (finely chopped) - 1 piece

Carrots (cut into matchsticks) - 1/2 cup

Peas (fresh or frozen) - 1/2 cup

Celery (chopped) - 2 stalks

Mushroom seasoning (powdered) - 2 tbsp

Chicken broth (fat-free) - 2 cups

Sour cream (fat-free, at room temp) - 1 cup

Garlic (minced) - 3 cloves

Salt (1 tsp)

Pepper (1/2 tsp)

Instructions

1.   Combine all **Ingredients** in a crockpot except the sour cream.

2.   For 4- 6 hrs., cook on low heat.

3.   For about 5 minutes, stir in sour cream, and warm until it is thoroughly heated. Serve immediately.

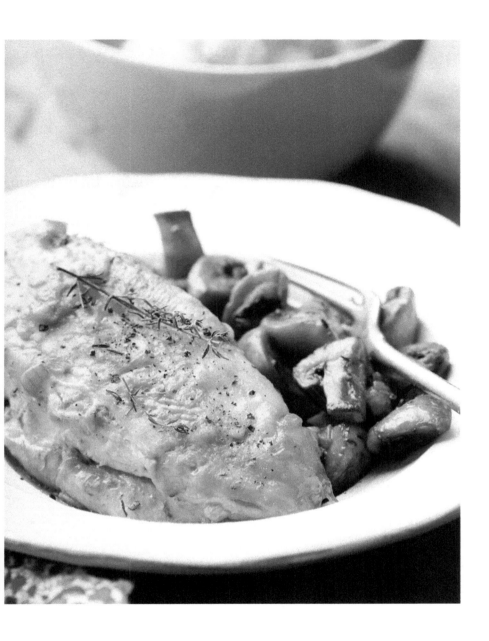

Smashed Avocado and Egg Toast

SmartPoints value: Green plan – 6SP, Blue plan – 4SP, Purple plan - 4SP

Total Time: 7 min, Prep time: 5 min, Cooking time: 2 min, Serves: 1

Nutritional value: Calories – 214.0, Carbs - 16.4g, Fat – 14.2g, Protein - 8.4g

Ingredients

Avocado - ¼ item(s), medium-sized, ripe but still a touch firm

Light whole-grain bread - 1 slice(s)

Whole hard-boiled egg(s) - 1 item(s), sliced

Table salt - 1 pinch

Crushed red pepper flakes - 1 pinch

Black pepper - 1 pinch

Instructions

1.   Place one slice of bread on a clean plate.

2.   Top with a portion of peeled avocado and gently smash with a knife or fork.

3.   Cut hard-boiled egg in half and place each half on the bread.

4.   Gently smash egg and mix with smashed avocado. Season the bread to taste with salt, pepper, and red pepper flakes.

5.   Cover with another slice of bread and place in a flat-sitting electric bread toaster.

6.   Remove smashed avocado and egg toast from the toaster once the "ready" light comes on.

Sweet Pineapple and Strawberry Salsa with Yogurt

The best salsas sometimes don't contain tomatoes, and this sweet pineapple and strawberry salsa with yogurt recipe is a good example.

I've added coconut flakes to this recipe to give a pleasant taste of fresh fruit.

SmartPoints value: Green plan – 3SP, Blue plan – 2SP, Purple plan - 2SP Total Time: 8 min, Prep time: 4 min, Cooking time: 4 min Serves: 1 Nutritional value: Calories - 30.9, Carbs - 7.4g, Fat - 0.4g, Protein - 0.4g

Ingredients

Strawberries - 3 medium-sized, diced - fresh mint leaves - 1 tsp (chopped)

Pineapple - ½ cup(s), Golden species (diced)

Plain fat-free Greek yogurt - ½ cup(s)

Lime zest - ⅛ tsp (grated)

Unsweetened coconut flakes - 1 Tbsp (toasted)

Coconut flakes – 3 Tbsp

Instructions

Dice strawberries, pineapple, mint, and lime zest into a small bowl, all mixed.

Add yogurt and speckle with coconut. You can also spoon the yogurt into a glass dish and top it with fruit and coconut.

Creamy Banana French Toast Casserole

You can give a bright flavor to this creamy casserole and also keep the banana from turning black by adding a small quantity of lemon juice.

SmartPoints value: Green plan – 7SP, Blue plan – 6SP, Purple plan - 6SP

Total Time: 55 min, Prep time: 20 min, Cooking time: 35 min, Serves: 12

Nutritional value:

Calories - 489, Carbs - 68.7g, Fat - 18g, Protein - 15.4g

Ingredients

Cooking spray - 5 spray(s)

Whole wheat/oatmeal bread - 12 slice(s), cut into quarters (about 1 oz per slice)

Neufchâtel cheese - 4 oz, (1/3-less-fat cream cheese)

2% reduced-fat milk - 1 cup(s)

Maple syrup - ½ cup(s)

Egg(s) - 6 large

Banana(s) - 4 medium-sized, ripe (divided)

Fresh lemon juice - 2 tsp

Rum - 1 Tbsp

Ground cinnamon - ½ tsp

Vanilla extract - 1 tsp

Ground nutmeg - ½ tsp

Table salt - ¼ tsp

Powdered sugar - 3 Tbsp

Instructions

1.   Get a clean 13 inches by 9 inches baking dish and coat it with cooking spray.

2.   Stand quarter portions of bread up in the prepared dish, so it lines the sides and bottom in a single layer — Preheat the oven to 350°F.

3.   Place the cheese, milk, and syrup in a blender.

4.   Add eggs, two bananas, rum, vanilla, juice, nutmeg, cinnamon, and salt to the blender.

5.   Allow the blending process to Dash until the mixture is smooth.

6.   Gently pour the mixture over the bread and press those on the sides of the baking dish into the egg mixture, making sure it is completely submerged.

7.   Refrigerate the dish for 30 minutes after covering with foil.

8.   Preheat the oven again to 350°F. Just before baking, thinly slice the remaining two bananas and put the slices in between pieces of bread.

9.   Cover the dish with new foil and bake for 25 minutes. Remove the foil and continue baking until the color is golden brown. Set for about 10 minutes more, then sprinkle the top with powdered sugar. Slice the casserole into 12 pieces and serve immediately.

Fried Egg with Asparagus-Potato Hash

SmartPoints value: Green plan – 7SP, Blue plan – 5SP, Purple plan - 1SP Total Time: 22 min, Prep time: 12 min, Cooking time: 10 min, Serves: 1 Nutritional value: Calories - 319, Carbs - 38.4g, Fat - 8g, Protein - 11.5g

Ingredients

Uncooked red potato(es) - 1 medium-sized, pierced severally with a fork

Uncooked asparagus - 4 spear(s), medium-sized, trimmed, diagonally sliced 1/2-inch thick (1/2 cup)

Uncooked scallion(s) - 1 small (sliced)

Olive oil - 1 tsp

Table salt - ¼ tsp

Fresh thyme - 1 tsp (chopped)

Egg(s) - 1 large, cooked sunny-side up

Black pepper - 1 pinch

Instructions

1. Microwave potato for about 3-4 minutes and cut into smal
dice.

2. Heat the oil in a medium-sized, nonstick skillet over a
medium to high heat.

3. Add the asparagus and diced potato to the oil

4. Cook, occasionally stirring, until the diced potatoes are
browned, and asparagus is crisp-tender, about 4 minutes.

5. Add the scallion and thyme; keep stirring until scallior
wilts, about 30 seconds.

6. Season with salt and pepper, then serve with egg.

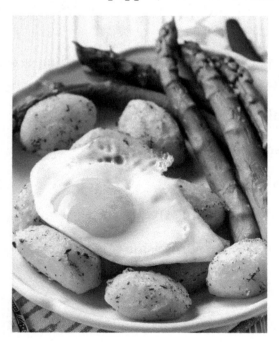

Greek-Style Scrambled Eggs

If you need a quick and easy weeknight dish, you can prepare these scrambled eggs within 20 minutes. These eggs make a perfect one-dish meal, loaded with various flavors that include butter beans, chicken chorizo sausage, grape tomatoes, and onions.

To make this meal vegetarian, add soy-based breakfast sausage. You can use lentils in place of butter beans if you can't find them.

Prevent overcooking by turning off the heat before the eggs are all the way cooked.

SmartPoints value: Green plan – 8SP, Blue plan – 3SP, Purple plan - 3SP Total Time: 20 min, Prep time: 12 min, Cooking time: 8 min, Serves: 1 Nutritional value: Calories - 221, Carbs - 5.1g, Fat - 10.3g, Protein - 21.0g

Ingredients

Cooked chicken chorizo sausage - 1½ oz (diced)

Cooking spray - 5 spray(s)

Canned butter beans - ¼ cup(s), rinsed and drained

Crumbled feta cheese - 1 Tbsp

Uncooked onion(s) - ¼ cup(s) (chopped)

Grape tomatoes - 6 medium-sized (halved)

Egg(s) - 2 large

Black pepper - 1 pinch, or add to taste

Table salt - 1 pinch, or add to taste

Dill - 1 Tbsp, chopped

Instructions

1.   Coat a medium-sized nonstick skillet with nonstick spray.

2.   Add chicken chorizo and onion, then cook over medium heat, occasionally stirring, until lightly browned, about 5 minutes.

3.   Add tomatoes and beans, then stir until the tomatoes start to soften, about 1 minute.

4.   Push the mixture to one side of the skillet and add eggs to the other side.

5.   Scramble the eggs until softly set, 1-2 minutes.

6.   Turn in the chorizo mixture and season with salt and pepper, then sprinkle with dill and feta.

Black Bean Vegan Wraps

Nutritional Facts

servings per container	5
Prep Total	**10 min**
Serving Size 2/3 cup (27g)	
Amount per serving **Calories**	**200**
	% Daily Value
Total Fat 8g	1%
Saturated Fat 1g	2%
Trans Fat 0g	2%
Cholesterol	**2%**
Sodium 240mg	7%
Total Carbohydrate 12g	**2%**
Dietary Fiber 4g	14%
Total Sugar 12g	01.21%
Protein 3g	
Vitamin C 2mcg	2%
Calcium 20mg	1%
Iron 7mg	2%
Potassium 25mg	6%

Ingredients

1 1/2 half cup of beans (sprouted & cooked)

2 carrot

1 or 2 tomatoes

2 avocados

1 cob of corn

1 Kale

2 or 3 sticks of celery

2 persimmons

1 Coriander

Dressing:

1 hachiyapersimmon (or half a mango)

Juice of 1 lemon

2 to 3 tablespoons original olive oil

1/4 clean cup water

1 or 2 teaspoons grated fresh ginger

1/2 teaspoon of salt

Instructions:

1.   Sprout & cook the black beans

2.   Chop all the **Ingredients** & mix them in a neat bowl with the black beans

3.   Mix all the **Ingredients** for the dressing & pour into the salad

4.   Serve a spoonful in a clean lettuce leaf that you can easily roll into a wrap. Most people do use iceberg or romaine lettuce.

Fascinating Spinach and Beef Meatballs

Serving: 4

Prep Time: 10 minutes

Cook Time: 20

Ingredients:

½ cup onion

4 garlic cloves

1 whole egg

¼ teaspoon oregano

Pepper as needed

1-pound lean ground beef

10 ounces spinach

How To:

1.   Preheat   your   oven   to   375   degrees   F.
2.   Take a bowl and blend within the remainder of the **Ingredients**, and using your hands, roll into meatballs.

3.   Transfer to a sheet tray and bake for 20 minutes.

4.   Enjoy!

Nutrition (Per Serving)

Calorie: 200
Fat: 8g
Carbohydrates: 5g
Protein: 29g

Juicy and Peppery Tenderloin

Serving: 4

Prep Time: 10 minutes

Cook Time: 20

Ingredients:

2 teaspoons sage, chopped

Sunflower seeds and pepper

2 1/2 pounds beef tenderloin

2 teaspoons thyme, chopped

2 garlic cloves, sliced

2 teaspoons rosemary, chopped

4 teaspoons olive oil

How To:

1.   Preheat your oven to 425 degrees F.

2.   Take alittle knife and cut incisions within the tenderloin; insert one slice of garlic into the incision.

3.   Rub meat with oil.

4.   Take a bowl and add sunflower seeds, sage, thyme, rosemary, pepper and blend well.

5.   Rub the spice mix over tenderloin.

6.   Put rubbed tenderloin into the roasting pan and bake for 10 minutes.

7.   Lower temperature to 350 degrees F and cook for 20 minutes more until an indoor thermometer reads 145 degrees F.

8.   Transfer tenderloin to a chopping board and let sit for 15 minutes; slice through 20 pieces and enjoy!

Nutrition (Per Serving)

Calorie: 183

Fat: 9g

Carbohydrates: 1g

Protein: 24g

Healthy Avocado Beef Patties

Serving: 2

Prep Time: 15 minutes

Cook Time: 10 minutes

Ingredients

1 pound 85% lean ground beef
1 small avocado, pitted and peeled
Fresh ground black pepper as needed

How To:

1. Pre-heat and prepare your broiler to high.
2. Divide beef into two equal-sized patties.
3. Season the patties with pepper accordingly.
4. Broil the patties for five minutes per side.
5. Transfer the patties to a platter.
6. Slice avocado into strips and place them on top of the patties.
7. Serve and enjoy!

Nutrition (Per Serving)
Calories: 568
Fat: 43g
Net Carbohydrates: 9g
Protein: 38g

Ravaging Beef Pot Roast

Serving: 4

Prep Time: 10 minutes

Cook Time: 75 minutes

Ingredients:

3 ½ pounds beef roast

4 ounces mushrooms, sliced

12 ounces beef stock

1-ounce onion soup mix

½ cup Italian dressing, low sodium, and low fat

How To:

1.   Take a bowl and add the stock, onion soup mix and Italian dressing.

2.   Stir.

3.   Put roast beef in pan.

4.   Add mushrooms, stock mix to the pan and canopy with foil.

5.   Preheat your oven to 300 degrees F.

6.   Bake for 1 hour and quarter-hour .

7.   Let the roast cool.

8.   Slice and serve.

9.   Enjoy with the gravy on top!

Nutrition (Per Serving)

Calories: 700

Fat: 56g

Carbohydrates: 10g

Protein: 70g

Rainbow Nourishment Bowl

Nutritional Facts

servings per container	5
Prep Total	**10 min**
Serving Size 2/3 cup (77g)	
Amount per serving **Calories**	**20**
	% Daily Value
Total Fat 2g	**0%**
Saturated Fat 7g	2%
Trans Fat 0g	10%
Cholesterol	**5%**
Sodium 55mg	**20%**
Total Carbohydrate 9g	**200%**
Dietary Fiber 7g	1%
Total Sugar 36g	2%
Protein 1g	
Vitamin C 6mcg	21%
Calcium 160mg	2%
Iron 7mg	2%
Potassium 320mg	10%

Ingredients

2 cups spinach

1/2 cup corn kernels

1/2 cup edamame beans

1/2 cup cabbage, shredded

1/4 cup carrots, sliced

1/2 cup quinoa, cooked

1 radish, sliced

Handful pea shoot sprouts (or another type of sprouts)

1/2 avocado, sliced

Sesame seeds

Juice of 1/2 lemon

Instructions:

1.   Start by filling the bottom of the Coconut Bowls with spinach.

2.   Place the corn, edamame, cabbage, carrots, cooked quinoa, radish, sprouts, & avocado in small piles on top of the bowls.

3.   Sprinkle with sesame seeds.

4.   Dress with some lemon juice if desired

Caramelized Banana & Blueberry Tacos

Nutritional Facts

Serving per container	7
Prep total	10 min
Serving size 2/3 cup (51g)	
Amount per serving	11
Calories	
	% Daily Value
Total Fat 2g	**2%**
Saturated Fat 7g	10%
Trans Fat 3g	8%
Cholesterol	**9%**
Sodium 470mg	**2%**
Total Carbohydrate 20g	**200%**
Dietary Fiber 10g	20%
Total Sugar 9g	1%
Protein 6g	
Vitamin C 1mcg	20%
Calcium 700mg	7%
Iron 7mg	2%
Potassium 470mg	9%

Ingredients

4 flour tortillas

1 Teaspoon coconut oil

2 ripe bananas, peeled and sliced lengthways into 0.5cm / 0.2" slices

100g / 3.5oz fresh blueberries

1 Teaspoon maple syrup

3 Teaspoon vanilla favored coconut or soy yogurt

1 heaped teaspoon tahini

1.5 Teaspoon shredded coconut or coconut flakes

1 Teaspoon cacao nibs

Instructions:

1.   You will need to preheat the oven to 160°C / 320°F.

2.   Kindly wrap the tortillas in foil & heat in the oven for 6 minutes.

3.   Heat a medium-sized, heavy-based, non-stick or cast-iron skillet on medium heat on the stove. Add original coconut oil & once it's melted, add the sliced clean bananas.

4.   Fry the bananas until they are golden brown on both sides, making sure to rotate them frequently so they won't stick to the pan.

5.   You need to top the warm tortillas with the fried bananas and drizzle with tahini, yogurt, and maple syrup.

6.   Kindly top with blueberries and sprinkle with coconut and cacao nibs.

7.   Serve and enjoy

Decent Beef and Onion Stew

Serving: 4

Prep Time: 10 minutes

Cook Time 1-2 hours

Ingredients:

2 pounds lean beef, cubed

3 pounds shallots, peeled

5 garlic cloves, peeled, whole

3 tablespoons tomato paste

1 bay leaves

¼ cup olive oil

3 tablespoons lemon juice

How To:

1.   Take a stew pot and place it over medium heat.

2.   Add vegetable oil and let it heat up.

3.   Add meat and brown.

4.   Add remaining **Ingredients** and canopy with water.

5.   Bring the entire mix to a boil.

6.   Reduce heat to low and canopy the pot.

7.   Simmer for 1-2 hours until beef is cooked thoroughly.

8.   Serve hot!

Nutrition (Per Serving)

Calories: 136

Fat: 3g

Carbohydrates: 0.9g

Protein: 24g

Clean Parsley and Chicken Breast

Serving: 2

Prep Time: 10 minutes

Cook Time: 40 minutes

Ingredients:

1/2 tablespoon dry parsley

1/2 tablespoon dry basil

2 chicken breast halves, boneless and skinless 1/4 teaspoon sunflower seeds

1/4 teaspoon red pepper flakes, crushed 1 tomato, sliced

How To:

1.	Pre-heat your oven to 350 degrees F.

2.	Take a 9x13 inch baking dish and grease it up with cooking spray.

3.	Sprinkle 1 tablespoon of parsley, 1 teaspoon of basil and spread the mixture over your baking dish.

4.	Arrange the pigeon breast halves over the dish and sprinkle garlic slices on top.

5.	Take a little bowl and add 1 teaspoon parsley, 1 teaspoon of basil, sunflower seeds, basil, red pepper and blend well. Pour the mixture over the pigeon breast.

6.	Top with tomato slices and canopy, bake for 25 minutes.

7.	Remove the duvet and bake for quarter-hour more.

8.	Serve and enjoy!

Nutrition (Per Serving)

Calories: 150

Fat: 4g

Carbohydrates: 4g

Protein: 25g

Roasted Red Pepper and Tomato Soup

SmartPoints value: Green plan - 1SP, Blue plan - 1SP, Purple plan - 1SP

Total Time: 1hr 20min, Prep time: 10 min, Cooking time: 1hr 10mins,

Serves: 6

Nutritional value: Calories – 107, Carbs – 19.4g, Fat – 0.4g, Protein – 4g

Ingredients

Plum tomatoes - 10 pieces

Bell peppers (red) - 3 pieces

Onion - 1 small

Olive oil - 1 tbsp

Garlic - 4 cloves

Tomato paste - 1/4 cup

Apple cider vinegar - 3 tbsp

Paprika - 1 tsp

Oregano (dried) - 1 tsp

Thyme (dried) - 1 tsp

A small handful of basil

Desired salt and pepper to taste

Instructions

1.	With a cooking spray, line a large rimmed baking sheet and put it in an over 400 degrees preheated oven.

2.	Slice each tomato into four slices, remove the seeds inside the pepper and slice into eighths. Place the peppers, garlic cloves and tomatoes onto the prepared baking sheet and mist with an olive oil mister. Evenly sprinkle the paprika, oregano, thyme, and salt and pepper on top, then place in oven and roast for 30-35 minutes.

3.	In a large pot, heat the olive oil and add diced onions and sauté and leave until they begin to soften in about 2 minutes.

4.	Lower the heat and add roasted vegetables and garlic cloves, able cider vinegar, tomato paste, fresh basil, and two cups of water. Blend using the immersion blender until it gets smooth.

5.	Lower the heat further and add in the roasted vegetables and garlic cloves, tomato paste, able cider vinegar, fresh basil, and two cups of water, add water to achieve desired consistency.

6.	Add pepper and salt to taste and cover on low heat. Stir for about 20-30 minutes regularly.

7.   This homemade meal is sure to become your gateway. Savor the flavor of the roasted veggies and garlic.

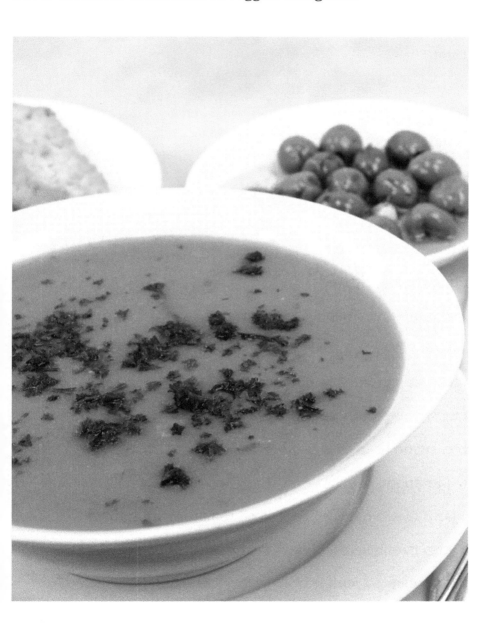

Black Bean-Tomato Chili

Total Time

Prep: 10 min. Cook: 35 min.

Makes

6 servings (2-1/4 quarts)

Ingredients:

2 tablespoons olive oil

1 huge onion, cleaved

1 medium green pepper, cleaved

3 garlic cloves, minced

1 teaspoon ground cinnamon

1 teaspoon ground cumin

1 teaspoon bean stew powder

1/4 teaspoon pepper

3 jars (14-1/2 ounces each) diced tomatoes, undrained

2 jars (15 ounces each) dark beans, washed and depleted

1 cup squeezed orange or juice from 3 medium oranges

Directions:

1.   In a Dutch broiler, heat oil over medium-high warmth. Include onion and green pepper; cook and mix 8-10 minutes or until delicate. Include garlic and seasonings; cook brief longer.

2.   Mix in residual fixings; heat to the point of boiling. Lessen heat; stew, secured, 20-25 minutes to enable flavors to mix, blending incidentally.

Mushroom & Broccoli Soup

Total Time

Prep: 20 min. Cook: 45 min.

Makes

8 servings

Ingredients:

1 bundle broccoli (around 1-1/2 pounds)

1 tablespoon canola oil

1/2 pound cut crisp mushrooms

1 tablespoon diminished sodium soy sauce

2 medium carrots, finely slashed

2 celery ribs, finely slashed

1/4 cup finely slashed onion

1 garlic clove, minced

1 container (32 ounces) vegetable juices

2 cups of water

2 tablespoons lemon juice

Directions:

1. Cut broccoli florets into reduced down pieces. Strip and hack stalks.

2. In an enormous pot, heat oil over medium-high warmth; saute mushrooms until delicate, 4-6 minutes. Mix in soy sauce; expel from skillet.

3. In the same container, join broccoli stalks, carrots, celery, onion, garlic, soup, and water; heat to the point of boiling. Diminish heat; stew, revealed, until vegetables are relaxed, 25-30 minutes.

4. Puree soup utilizing a drenching blender. Or then again, cool marginally and puree the soup in a blender; come back to the dish. Mix in florets and mushrooms; heat to the point of boiling. Lessen warmth to medium; cook until broccoli is delicate, 8-10 minutes, blending infrequently. Mix in lemon juice.

Avocado Fruit Salad with

Tangerine Vinaigrette

Total Time

Prep/Total Time: 25 min.

Makes

8 servings

Ingredients:

3 medium ready avocados, stripped and meagerly cut

3 medium mangoes, stripped and meagerly cut

1 cup crisp raspberries

1 cup crisp blackberries

1/4 cup minced crisp mint

1/4 cup cut almonds, toasted

Dressing:

1/2 cup olive oil

1 teaspoon ground tangerine or orange strip 1/4 cup tangerine or squeezed orange

2 tablespoons balsamic vinegar

1/2 teaspoon salt

1/4 teaspoon naturally ground pepper

Directions:

1.   Mastermind avocados and organic product on a serving plate; sprinkle with mint and almonds. In a little bowl, whisk dressing fixings until mixed; shower over a plate of mixed greens.

2.   To toast nuts, prepare in a shallow container in a 350° stove for 5-10 minutes or cook in a skillet over low warmth until softly sautéed, mixing every so often.

General Salad Cauliflower

Total Time

Prep: 25 min. Cook: 20 min.

Makes

4 servings

Ingredients:

Oil for profound fat fricasseeing

1/2 cup generally useful flour

1/2 cup cornstarch

1 teaspoon salt

1 teaspoon preparing powder

3/4 cup club pop

1 medium head cauliflower, cut into 1-inch florets (around 6 cups)

Sauce:

1/4 cup squeezed orange

3 tablespoons sugar

3 tablespoons soy sauce

3 tablespoons vegetable stock

2 tablespoons rice vinegar

2 teaspoons sesame oil

2 teaspoons cornstarch

2 tablespoons canola oil

2 to 6 dried pasilla or other hot chilies, cleaved

3 green onions, white part minced, green part daintily cut

3 garlic cloves, minced

1 teaspoon ground new gingerroot

1/2 teaspoon ground orange get-up-and-go 4 cups hot cooked rice

Directions:

1.   In an electric skillet or profound fryer, heat oil to 375°. Consolidate flour, cornstarch, salt, and heating powder. Mix in club soft drink just until mixed (hitter will be slender). Plunge florets, a couple at once, into the player and fry until cauliflower are delicate and covering is light dark colored, 8-10 minutes. Channel on paper towels.

2.   For the sauce, whisk together the initial six fixings; race n cornstarch until smooth.

3.   In a huge pot, heat canola oil over medium-high warmth. nclude chilies; cook and mix until fragrant, 2 minutes. Include

white piece of onions, garlic, ginger, and orange get-up-and-go cook until fragrant, around 1 moment. Mix soy sauce blend; add to the pan. Heat to the point of boiling; cook and mix until thickened, 4 minutes.

4.   Add cauliflower to sauce; hurl to cover. Present with rice; sprinkle with daintily cut green onions.

Salad Chickpea Mint Tabbouleh

Total Time

Prep/Total Time: 30 min.

Makes

4 servings

Ingredients:

1 cup bulgur

2 cups of water

1 cup new or solidified peas (around 5 ounces), defrosted

1 can (15 ounces) chickpeas or garbanzo beans, washed and depleted

1/2 cup minced new parsley

1/4 cup minced new mint

1/4 cup olive oil

2 tablespoons julienned delicate sun-dried tomatoes (not stuffed in oil)

2 tablespoons lemon juice

1/2 teaspoon salt

1/4 teaspoon pepper

Directions:

1.   In a huge pot, consolidate bulgur and water; heat to the point of boiling. Decrease heat; stew, secured, 10 minutes. Mix in crisp or solidified peas; cook, secured, until bulgur and peas are delicate, around 5 minutes.

2.   Move to an enormous bowl. Mix in outstanding fixings. Serve warm, or refrigerate and serve cold.

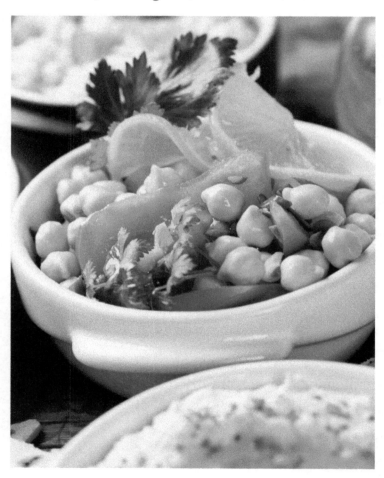

Creamy Cauliflower Pakora Soup

Total Time

Prep: 20 min. Cook: 20 min.

Makes

8 servings (3 quarts)

Ingredients:

1 huge head cauliflower, cut into little florets

5 medium potatoes, stripped and diced

1 huge onion, diced

4 medium carrots, stripped and diced

2 celery ribs, diced

1 container (32 ounces) vegetable stock

1 teaspoon garam masala

1 teaspoon garlic powder

1 teaspoon ground coriander

1 teaspoon ground turmeric

1 teaspoon ground cumin

1 teaspoon pepper

1 teaspoon salt

1/2 teaspoon squashed red pepper chips Water or extra vegetable stock New cilantro leaves

Lime wedges, discretionary

Directions

1.   In a Dutch stove over medium-high warmth, heat initial 14 fixings to the point of boiling. Cook and mix until vegetables are delicate, around 20 minutes. Expel from heat; cool marginally. Procedure in groups in a blender or nourishment processor until smooth. Modify consistency as wanted with water (or extra stock). Sprinkle with new cilantro. Serve hot, with lime wedges whenever wanted.

2.   Stop alternative: Before including cilantro, solidify cooled soup in cooler compartments. To utilize, in part defrost in cooler medium-term. Warmth through in a pan, blending every so often and including a little water if fundamental. Sprinkle with cilantro. Whenever wanted, present with lime wedges.

Spice Trade Beans and Bulgur

Total Time

Prep: 30 min. Cook: 3-1/2 hours

Makes

10 servings

Ingredients:

3 tablespoons canola oil, isolated

2 medium onions, slashed

1 medium sweet red pepper, slashed

5 garlic cloves, minced

1 tablespoon ground cumin

1 tablespoon paprika

2 teaspoons ground ginger

1 teaspoon pepper

1/2 teaspoon ground cinnamon

1/2 teaspoon cayenne pepper

1-1/2 cups bulgur

1 can (28 ounces) squashed tomatoes

1 can (14-1/2 ounces) diced tomatoes, undrained

1 container (32 ounces) vegetable juices

2 tablespoons darker sugar

2 tablespoons soy sauce

1 can (15 ounces) garbanzo beans or chickpeas, flushed and depleted

1/2 cup brilliant raisins

Minced crisp cilantro, discretionary

Directions:

1.   In an enormous skillet, heat 2 tablespoons oil over medium-high warmth. Include onions and pepper; cook and mix until delicate, 3-4 minutes. Include garlic and seasonings; cook brief longer. Move to a 5-qt. slow cooker.

2.   In the same skillet, heat remaining oil over medium-high warmth. Include bulgur; cook and mix until daintily caramelized, 2-3 minutes or until softly sautéed.

3.   Include bulgur, tomatoes, stock, darker sugar, and soy sauce to slow cooker. Cook, secured, on low 3-4 hours or until bulgur is delicate. Mix in beans and raisins; cook 30 minutes longer.

Whenever wanted, sprinkle with cilantro.

Tofu Chow Mein

Total Time

Prep: 15 min. + standing Cook: 15 min.

Makes

4 servings

Ingredients:

8 ounces uncooked entire wheat holy messenger hair pasta

3 tablespoons sesame oil, separated

1 bundle (16 ounces) extra-firm tofu

2 cups cut new mushrooms

1 medium sweet red pepper, julienned

1/4 cup decreased sodium soy sauce

3 green onions daintily cut

Directions:

1.   Cook pasta as per bundle headings. Channel; flush with cold water and channel once more. Hurl with 1 tablespoon oil; spread onto a preparing sheet and let remain around 60 minutes.

2.   In the meantime, cut tofu into 1/2-in. 3D shapes and smudge dry. Enclose by a spotless kitchen towel; place on a plate and refrigerate until prepared to cook.

3.   In an enormous skillet, heat 1 tablespoon oil over medium warmth. Include pasta, spreading equitably; cook until base is daintily caramelized, around 5 minutes. Expel from skillet.

4.   In the same skillet, heat remaining oil over medium-high warmth; pan sear mushrooms, pepper, and tofu until mushrooms are delicate, 3-4 minutes. Include pasta and soy sauce; hurl and warmth through. Sprinkle with green onions.

Broiled Tilapia

SmartPoints value: Green plan - 2SP, Blue plan - 0SP, Purple plan - 0SP

Total Time: 13 min, Prep time: 8 min, Cooking time: 5 min, Serves: 4

Nutritional value: Cal - 154.8, Carbs - 1.5g, Fat - 6.4g, Protein - 22.8g

You can apply this recipe with other types of fish, such as sole, halibut, flounder, and even shellfish. You also swap lime juice for lemon juice.

Ingredients

Black pepper - ¼ tsp, freshly ground

Cooking spray - 1 spray(s)

Garlic (herb seasoning) - 2 tsp

Lemon juice (fresh) - 1 Tbsp

Table salt - ½ tsp (or to taste)

Tilapia fillet(s) (uncooked) - 20 oz, four 5 oz fillets

Instructions

1.   Prepare your grill by preheating. Coat a skillet with cooking spray.

2.   Apply seasoning to both sides of the fish with salt and pepper.

3.   Transfer the fish to the prepared skillet and drizzle it with lemon juice, then sprinkle garlic herb seasoning over the top.

4.   Broil the fish until it is fork-tender; about 5 minutes.